"If we could give every individual the right amount of nourishment and exercise, not too little and not too much, we would have found the safest way to health!"

Hippocrates (circa 400 BC)

Distributed by:

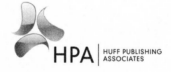

Cover Design by:

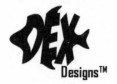

Well Planet

Fitness as a Spiritual Discipline

Well Planet

Fitness as a Spiritual Discipline

Part I
Hacking at the Leaves

Call Me Hope

You would have called me fat twelve years ago. You would have seen me from a distance and whispered to someone, "Wow she is fat!" Or worse, you might have just pointed. I could sense when people whispered or pointed even if I wasn't looking at them directly. It broke me down a bit. But the ironic thing is it never moved me to do something to fix it. Oh don't get me wrong, I dieted, lost, and then gained, then lost. I tried shakes and pills and everything in between. But, being fat made me think of being skinny all the time. Now, years later, I am in shape and I don't think about being fat or skinny or anything. I just am.

I have found that making efforts to be in good shape is now like brushing teeth or showering, you just do it without the hassle of thinking about it. It is just a part of me, part of my routine. If I miss brushing my teeth, my mouth feels gross. When I miss a shower, my skin feels gross as well. I do those things because they make me feel better. Running makes me feel better. Eating healthy makes me feel better. I really eat healthy and exercise because the long term benefits will make my life much easier. But really, in the short term, I just want to feel better.

Exercise literally pressure washes your body clean from the inside out. Sweat and a rapid increase in blood flow carry away stagnant impurities and toxins, initiating an orchestra of physical healing. Even if you aren't aware of this, you feel it.

After exercising you just feel cleaner and better, like after brushing your teeth or taking a shower.

Call me Hope. This is the name my parents gave me the day I arrived into this world fifty-seven years ago. What you need to know about me is that twelve years ago, I was in a dark place. I was not always as happy as I am now.

I thought life was over for me at forty-five. I didn't talk about it for a long time, but I do now. I was talked into telling my story by one of my best friends, who happens to be a one-hundred year old monk. Yep, a century old wise holy man is one of my best friends. He put me up to telling my whole story through those dark years. He says I owe it to readers to tell it. He says some readers might be in the same dark place. So I am writing down my story.

This book isn't so much about me as much as it is about what I have learned from my old monk friend, Brother Mark. So, if he is right and you are in a similar place where I was twelve years ago before I met him, he has so much he can teach you too.

On our first meeting, he and I visited for four hours. I was no longer in the dark after we met. It won't take you as long to see the light. You will most likely finish reading this short book in a lot less than four hours.

I will assume you are reading this because you might want some help getting healthy; maybe you are one who struggles like I did. Well then, I hope this story lives up to what Brother Mark is hoping for you. He feels my message is good enough to save you from taking the same miserable fall that I almost took before he "caught" me from going off a cliff. Not a literal cliff, but a cliff as a metaphor meaning despair, or death, or something.

I always look to Brother Mark as being like the Holden Caulfield character in the J. D. Salinger book *The Catcher in the Rye*. As depressingly sad as the book was when I had to read it in high school, the image of "catching" innocent children playing in the rye grass before they fell off a cliff is a pretty powerful image. In case you don't know the book, that is what the *Catcher* is according to Salinger. The Catcher stands at the edge of the cliff while innocent children, who are completely unaware of the danger, play in the nearby rye grass. His awareness of the cliff saves the children from falling to their death, or their despair, or something.

I will always see Brother Mark as my catcher. Without him, I would have fallen. I might even have jumped, who knows. However, he caught me and saved me, both physically and spiritually, I would say.

Before I get too far ahead of myself, let me get you up to speed. None of this story will make any sense unless I bring you back to that day twelve years ago to my first encounter with the monk and the four hours that saved my life.

Twelve Years Ago

I remember the day was a fall day. Fall is an incredible season in eastern Pennsylvania. It contains the days where, after three months of hot summer sun and stickiness, you can walk barefoot in the cool grass. These fall days are perfect! The day I met Brother Mark the humidity was completely lifted and there was the distinct smell of freshly cut hay from the miles of surrounding farms. There was even an occasional *whiff* of farm animals depending on the wind direction; and to be quite honest, even that was pleasant. It seems nothing connects me to nature like the smell of fresh earth on a cool fall day in one of the greenest valleys of rolling hills in America. You appreciate the surrounding beauty even more when you realize that the Amish people of the area have always treaded lightly on this part of the planet. Most people know of the Amish, not only for their horses and buggies, but for the fact that they farm the old fashion way. They farm like everyone did for hundreds of years before conventional chemicals, tractors, and diesel fuel.

The greenery, the smells, and the fresh air are all a direct result of centuries of the Amish working the soil on the west side of this valley - the *Lehigh Valley*. In case you don't know, the Lehigh Valley is the region in Pennsylvania where the Lehigh River runs through it. It is just north of Philadelphia.

Organic farming is practiced here; not because it is trendy to not use pesticides, insecticides, and chemical fertilizers; but because this land and her Amish people have never chosen any other way to farm. The area is unspoiled. It is as if God said to conventional technology, *"Not here, the western side of this valley is reserved for these people who choose to continue to tread lightly on my land."*

This place is pristine and special because of the Amish, but it is also special because of the oldest religious community sitting in the center of the valley. The community's beautiful stone buildings are the homestead and workplace of many elderly monks of Saint Leo's Monastery. This community is a little different for this area because it is not an Amish community but a Catholic one. It is one of the oldest monasteries in the United States and is known for its hospitality. It serves as a spiritual center for many contemporary pilgrims who make their way to visit its resident brothers. This pilgrimage has been a tradition since the 18th century. Many holy men have walked its stone floors over the past two-hundred plus years.

Of all the current resident monks at this monastery, one in particular was and still is most known. He is Brother Mark O'Reilly. He is most known because he has a practical mission that has become quite popular. His mission is teaching each visitor, fitness as a spiritual discipline.

Because of his former career as a family practice physician, Brother Mark has fallen into this renowned role of *healer*, restoring health to the masses, one student at a time. Many come to see him to soak up his wisdom and to warm-up in his glow.

Twelve years ago on that fantastic fall day when I came to pay Brother Mark my first visit, I was oblivious to the beautiful surrounding landscapes outside because I was battling something dark and ugly inside me. It was as if something unholy - a demon perhaps - had stolen my happiness and my hope for a healthy future.

When I was sitting with him for the first time, I remember I was not just crying, I was *wailing*. I remember releasing all the pain of a lifetime of poor health because of my poor choices. I wailed for the diagnosis I had received just a few days before - the diagnosis of *heart disease*.

My tears dampened the paper I gripped tightly in my hand that I brought to show Brother Mark. It was my cardiogram results from earlier in the week. The scribbling on the paper was from my cardiologist who said I had a "weakened heart." My doctor explained it was a weakness brought on by years of abnormal physical stress and medications. He said I had a stable heart, but weakened all the same. He also told me I was a borderline diabetic and I really should be on high blood pressure medication. I had also been treated for bouts of depression in the past. So I wailed—for my children, for my husband, and for myself. I wailed for all the disappointments in my forty-five years of living. I had lived preoccupied, living to be skinny, but never fully living. The culmination of the years of crazy fad diets, the medications, the stress, and the desperation threatened to take away what years I had left. So I wailed for it all.

About one year before that first day at the monastery, a colleague of mine at the Elementary School where I am a teacher, had suggested I travel to St. Leo's and visit with Brother Mark. The colleague had experienced firsthand the simple wisdom of this religious sage. I had been reluctant to make the trip, but my hesitancy to travel the fifty miles from Philadelphia to the monastery had finally been overcome because of my diagnosis. I was desperate, thus I finally made the pilgrimage to meet him.

"Why me?" I lamented to the elderly monk who I just met, who sat patiently next to me on a bench inside the monastery walls just outside of the *refectory* or dining hall where the monks gather for meals.

I remember Brother Mark gave no verbal response, only a deep look of concern. At eighty-eight years old, his face had a clear and youthful appearance (He really hasn't changed much over the twelve years since our first visit. He still has a clear and youthful appearance now at one-hundred years old).

During that first visit I remember saying to him a stream of pathetic statements, "I give up. I'm lost. I can't try anymore, I'm just so tired."

I remember there was still no response from Brother Mark. He continued to sit silent while holding my hand as I poured myself out to him.

I need to pause a moment and tell you a little more about my monk friend before I go on telling about that first encounter or else it won't make as much sense to you.

Farmer, Doctor, Monk

Brother Mark O'Reilly was once a physician at a time long before his life as a monk at St. Leo's. He was born and raised on a family farm in the western part of the Lehigh Valley not far from the monastery. He left briefly for Europe to fight in WWII, but eventually returned for medical school in Philadelphia. He graduated, married, and took up permanent residency in the farming village where he grew up.

His medical practice flourished for more than forty years. As a family physician, he cared for hundreds of children and their children and he became progressively more respected in his community as time went by. When it was time to retire, there was never such a celebration in the town as there was on behalf of the doctor and his wife. I was told the townspeople shut down the stores for the afternoon and young people came home from college. Even retirees flew back from their homes in Florida—all to celebrate the retirement of their doctor and his adored wife. The party was celebrated in the high school gymnasium and the local state congresswoman, a former lifelong patient, made the ninety

20

minute trip from Harrisburg to be the Master of Ceremonies. It made all the papers. The family physician had brought this farming community together simply by caring for its members.

The doctor and his wife retired by the Gulf of Mexico in the city of Fort Myers, Florida. They enjoyed several years on the beach, but then his wife's health slowly began to fail.

The doctor's deepest and fondest memories of those last weeks with her were sitting on the condo balcony watching sunsets on clear and beautiful evenings. Life had been good to both of them even though hers was cut short. They never had children. I don't know why. All these years, I never asked.

After the death of his beloved wife, after a year of grieving, he sold the condo, traveled to St. Leo's Monastery near his hometown in the Lehigh Valley in Pennsylvania, and at the age of seventy-five, the doctor joined the ranks of the other monks at the abbey and took the name "Brother Mark". He had lived there ever since.

Now that you know a little more about my friend, I can share with you more about my supernatural first encounter.

A Spiritual Path

After my meltdown, I remember sniffling and waiting for a response from Brother Mark. Along with the paper from my cardiologist, I was also clutching a wad of tissues to dab my runny nose and swollen eyes. I was empty, having withdrawn all of my emotional bank account with not even the strength left to ask him what he thought. We sat in silence while I allowed my hand to rest in the welcoming space of his hands. I remember I thought his thin and aged hands had a firm and calloused grip like a working man half his age.

The silence continued; but curiously, it was anything but awkward. I knew about Brother Mark for almost a year, but had only met him less than an hour before. I spent every ounce of energy I had, completely poured out my soul to him, and allowed my make-up to run without any effort to pull myself together. How odd, I thought. This same situation, at any other time in my life, would have made me extremely uncomfortable, because I wasn't confident enough to cry publicly or to be okay in silence with strangers.

The silence that day with Brother Mark was different than any other I had experienced. Somehow I felt peace just being held and supported. I wondered *why?* I didn't need to fill the silence with small talk. Despite the spectacle I had made of myself, I didn't feel embarrassment or shame. I felt something else; like a calming religious experience in a sense.

What made this time so different?

Brother Mark knew that my unhealthy situation was a much bigger problem. It was a national problem, not just my problem. I learned later that each year he had more and more unhealthy visitors. I wasn't the only one he "caught" from falling off the cliff. There were many of us he was a *Catcher* for, too many. He came to the conclusion years before the day of our meeting that no matter what efforts were made, it seemed nothing was striking at the root of the problem. People had been treating the symptoms, not the source. Over the years, I heard him quote a Henry David Thoreau line probably ten times: *"For every thousand hacking at the leaves of evil, there is one striking at the root."* He was referring to the diet pills, diet aids, fad diets, and other things that desperate visitors were trying - which was nothing more than profits for a weight-loss industry doomed to fail - maybe even *designed* to fail. All *were hacking at the leaves* and none getting at the root. If there wasn't failure of all these pills, powders, shakes, and fad diets, the multi-billion dollar a year diet industry would disappear. He knew this on our first meeting. I didn't know it at that point. Not yet.

I remember as I was pulling myself together, the wise monk leaned forward towards me and said, "I have, seen the strain of mounting health problems in our country from many struggling folks just like you Hope. Every story was as painful as the last. But all along, the simple solution to this problem is found by stepping back into a trusting relationship with our Creator."

I was not expecting those to be his first words to me after my breakdown. I was thinking that he would have lectured me on physical fitness or something because fitness was his thing. Instead, he was suggesting a spiritual solution. I was caught off guard, but also quite relieved. I was too tired to hear one more lecture from a doctor about how to lose weight. Those lectures obviously were not working.

His words made me feel good – relieved I guess. Quite frankly, I already knew that something deeper or more miraculous was going on that morning. I felt like our meeting was pre-destined somehow. All my life, I was missing a piece of the puzzle. I started to feel Brother Mark held that missing piece. I came into that monastery with the feeling that nothing could be done for me, that my fight for a healthy life had been lost. Now, in less than an hour, Brother Mark had started giving me hope. I didn't really know what to expect, I just knew it was different than all paths I went down before. I was in. Whatever spiritual path my new guru was leading me down, I was in.

A Simple Formula

I remember, after my meltdown we stood-up, stretched, and started walking down a well traveled path that surrounded the perimeter of the grounds of St. Leo's Monastery. The grounds were actually a good size working farm. I admit I started to finally notice the crispness in the air and the pleasant aromas of nature as we walked.

I continued to be surprised at just how comfortable I was in the monastery's silence. It made me wonder if I had ever *heard silence* before. I thought about the monks who lived in solitude on the grounds. They actually chose not to have the television on, not to have music blaring or anything filling the silence of their days other than the breeze in the trees, the birds singing, the free-range chickens *clucking*, and an occasional *moo* from their cattle, or *bah* from sheep in the distance.

It was nice. It was better than nice, it was somehow…

necessary, maybe? Without noisy distractions, I found myself

deeper in thought. I pondered things like cell phones.

Cell phones are a convenience, certainly; but they

seemed to be a constant technological distraction, just like

television. Without the distractions I was thinking more

clearly in the silence. Methodically, I began to calculate a

simple and disciplined approach to my weight and health

issues. I knew if I chose to eat a few less empty calories daily

and burned just a few more calories each day - without doing

anything else - I would be lighter, healthier. It was just simple

laws of physics and physiology. I started to remember a basic

formula buried somewhere in one of the older diet books I

had on my shelf back home:

Calories in < Calories out = Weight loss

That was the simple formula I remembered reading many, many years ago before that first visit.

In the heightened state of awareness I was in at the monastery, I started understanding how eating got so confusing. Eating healthy was simple but then I started to read the experts and all their diet books. The experts quickly scrambled the simple formula in my head. The experts taught me that I could only eat one type of food, which didn't seem to make sense to me, but I did it anyway. Then I starved myself according to the next expert. Other experts told me to eat only at certain times. I reduced my fats, then my carbohydrates, and finally my proteins. The experts sold me unnatural powders, shakes, and bars that didn't resemble food at all. Later, other experts warned against these unnatural bars, shakes, and powders. I was told to eat according to my blood type and my body type. All the diets had their successes, until I quit following them. In time, I gained my weight back and then some.

After a decade of struggling with this confusion, I decided to turn to more desperate measures. Despite warnings, I tried diet medications which were later pulled from the market. I tried various over-the-counter appetite suppressants. All failed in time. All failed to sustain a lifetime of health because I simply could not sustain it.

All of that came to me in that short time during that silent stroll with Brother Mark along the monastery perimeter following my meltdown. I remember we arrived at the door of the old stone building on the other side of the complex where that path ended. It was a small wooden door with an engraved name plate at eye level, one word surrounded by a border that resembled a crown of thorns: *Library*.

"Won't you step inside?" Brother Mark broke his silence.

Inside was a quaint little library. I expected just religious books, but there were books representing many genres: religion, farming, carpentry, botany, geography, and *wellness*. I was surprised. The books on the shelf marked for wellness were some of the same "Diet" books I had on my shelf at the time.

I remember after commenting on them, Brother Mark said the authors of those diet books had good intentions when they wrote their ideas down. Each felt they would solve the mounting health issues, yet the diet industry continued to thrive because no permanent cures had really been offered.

"The authors were forever treating the symptoms, never getting to the root of the problem. They are only hacking at the leaves, never striking at the root," this was the first time I remember hearing him use the Thoreau quote.

I asked him if he had read all of those diet books.

"Yes, I have," he answered.

"Why?" I was genuinely interested in why an eighty-eight year old retired doctor in remarkably good shape for his age would read diet books.

He answered by reminiscing about a time not so long ago when the weight-loss industry was non-existent. In fact, weight was almost never a problem for anyone when he was a young doctor, at least in his farming community. The growing epidemics of diabetes, high blood pressure, obesity, depression, cancer, and heart disease piqued his interest and lead him to read diet books. He wasn't looking for a cure so much as just investigating how far from the cure he felt experts were getting.

"Hope, today's crisis wasn't a crisis at all just a couple generations ago," Brother Mark continued, "Chronic health issues looked nothing like this when I was young. The problem was gradual. It crept up, disguised as *progress in the food industry*."

I did not know what he meant by this, but I was more than ready to learn.

Disturbing Statistic

While we were still in the library, Brother Mark mentioned the healthiest people on the planet were from Okinawa, Japan. They had a fraction of the heart disease and types of cancer we had in America and they were the longest living disability-free humans on the planet. He said they lived a lot like the Amish and like he did as a kid in rural America. As farmers, Okinawans worked very physical labor and fresh vegetables and healthy whole grains were the staple food they grew and ate.

He handed a book to me. It was a geography book about the Orient. The book was opened to a picture of a village in Okinawa. The picture was of a primitive farmer carrying buckets of what looked like assorted vegetables across a bamboo bridge, towards a cluster of huts. Women were gathering and preparing meals for the community.

I learned that the communities of rural Okinawa were not wealthy. They had no solid health care system, yet they possessed something greater. They had a clear and impassioned duty to the community. By individual villagers taking care of themselves, they could better care for others, especially the ones who are most vulnerable – children and seniors. They did this with a deep respect for their mother earth. According to Brother Mark, this was a lot like the early agricultural age in America before things started to change.

At that point in the meeting, I remember something really started to intensify the conversation. I didn't know if it was me thinking of how beautiful it would be to live in a community that was truly impassioned to provide for every member, or the fact I was so terribly unaware of the injustice of what Brother Mark was about to say next.

"In a world where nearly a billion people are starving," Brother Mark sighed, "We have about the same number of people who are overweight, obese, or *over* nourished."

I remember feeling very uncomfortable at that statistic. That was a dozen years ago and it still makes me shudder at the injustice. I knew immediately I was one of the billion who had too much food and certainly I did nothing to help the people who had no food. I was only focused on my personal "over-nourishment" all those years I was taking medications to stop my mindless eating. The same medications that made my heart weaken.

The planet has nearly a billion people who physically suffer for having too much, while a billion have next to nothing. This is what made my stomach start to turn.

Can all of us, the billion who eat too much, really have been that blind to the needs of the ones who had nothing to eat? Their hunger problem made my self-inflicted weight problem seem horribly selfish.

I felt the problem was hopeless for the poor because the self-centeredness of people like me who have resources but focus only on our own issues. A hungry billion is just too big a number.

Brother Mark assured me the poor's situation isn't hopeless. He said, "It does get better for the poor, one village at a time. It only seems too big a problem when we see one billion hungry people all at once; but, one village at a time - there is steady and sustainable hope."

He went on to explain some of the brothers at the monastery had been missionaries in third world countries. They had collected many stories of hopeless situations in villages with great poverty. In time, these villages were able to establish food cooperatives and were able to finally network their goods to consumers. Communities eventually started to get a foot on the rung of the ladder of sustainability. They were able to eat on a regular basis by using their own resources and sell the excess healthy crops to consumers for a sustainable profit. This was not just a feeding program that left a village dependent on support. This was something that kept a village fed through its own efforts. By teaching basic resourceful farming techniques, well digging and seed harvesting, these simple advancements turned the communities to sustainability one village at a time.

He explained everything from a water supply, to healthy crops, modest housing, education, healthcare, and gainful employment; all were accomplished with just a handful of able bodies who were willing to get the ball rolling for others.

"Thanks to a few people caring for others, the villagers could start to hack at the root of poverty, not the leaves." This was the second time I remember Brother Mark used a version of the Thoreau quote.

To be honest, it was his thoughtfulness that gave me mixed emotions. Initially, I was with him, enthusiastically hopeful. Then, I felt a tremendous paralyzing shame. His goodness really exposed my self-centeredness. My shame was because my whole life had been consumed on my single personal issue. My shallow health problem was exposed by the larger context of the world's food problem. My eyes were closed to the greater needs of others. I was feeling quite physically ill at that moment. I really was. I was trying to remember at what point in my life did I become blind to the needs of the starving billion? When did this madness of my obsession of my weight start to take over? When did my demon start speaking to me?

I need to pause again from the story and share a little more of my personal history so you can fully understand the shame I was feeling during that first visit.

Back to the Start

I was born, Elizabeth Hope Schaefer, into a caring middle class family from Philadelphia, Pennsylvania fifty-seven years ago. I attended public school and occasionally church and Sunday school. If asked, I would say I had a wonderful childhood. My parents were loving people. Always careful about where I went to play, when I came home, and what I ate. "Clean your plate and then you will get dessert," was the mantra that was said at dinner by my parents. My mother was a magnificently caring, moderately rotund woman who used her kitchen like a canvas. She was an artist with a spatula and a mixer, creating new dishes and baked goods that were mosaics of every cookbook and recipe she found. The memories and fragrances that came from my mother's kitchen, I will never forget. Today, if someone was grilling onions for *Philly Cheese Steak Sandwiches*, I instantly felt ten years old again. On Sunday afternoons after church sitting at the counter in our kitchen before the Eagles football game, my father and I would watch the food artist whip up her own recipe from scratch - a cheese steak calzone with homemade crust to be eaten during the game. There was great comfort in her food.

I never thought my weight was a problem as a child. I remember only once or twice in elementary school gym class when I was asked to climb a rope. I could not really even keep my feet off the ground for more than a few seconds. It just seemed strange that so many kids were climbing, some very well. The boys laughed at the fact that I didn't even get off the ground; but they were boys, they didn't count. I didn't care about boys anyway, none of the girls did yet. Not until middle school. It was in middle school when all things changed.

I remember like it was yesterday. I was with my very best girl friends at the first dance of the year in eighth grade. We were chatting near the refreshment table. The four of us girls did everything together. We made a pact to go to the same college and someday marry four boys who were best friends so we could all spend the rest of our lives together having sleepovers, eating popcorn, and watching movies. Yes, life was simple then. We had it all planned out.

It was *Devlin Hertz* who was walking towards our foursome at the dance. He was the middle school 'bad-boy' who wore a leather jacket all year long, not just when it was cold. He was one of the few eighth graders who rode a bicycle to school and was he handsome! All four of us girls thought so. I started to have a crush on him at the end of seventh grade. He never paid attention to me but that was normal. Most boys paid little attention to the girls they liked or who liked them. That was part of the hunt. It was as if the boys got together in the locker room and said to each other, "You like so and so - whatever you do, don't pay attention to her, and she will like you back." Boys were stupid at that age. If they only knew that the one thing girls talked about in eighth grade was them. Devlin Hertz was the one I talked about. I was smitten.

So there we were at the dance, Devlin approached us where we were standing by the punch and cookies, and asked "do you want to dance?" I swooned and said, "Me?"

Devlin responded with, "not you, her," as he pointed to Julia, one of the friends in our foursome. This was incredibly awkward for both Julia and me. Julia was well aware of the crush I had for Devlin. She looked nervously at me and then turned to Devlin.

"Okay...sure. I will dance with you Devlin," was all she said.

I felt the cold steel of the blade my best friend stuck in my back. But what Devlin uttered next pushed the blade in deeper to kill off any remaining dignity I had left. He said to me, "You stay here and guard the cookies, but save some for the rest of us." Then he laughed. I can still hear his laugh. They headed out to the dance floor together for a slow dance that only two other couples had the guts to dance to.

I was crushed. It took me weeks to recover, and a month before I talked to Julia. I never talked to Devlin Hertz again, although the thought of him somehow never left me, ever.

The morning after that dreadful night so long ago, I remember approaching my father to ask him a serious question. I know he would tell me what he thought would make me feel good. However this time, I hoped my dad would be painfully honest with me.

"Tell me not what I want to hear but the truth." I cleared my throat, "Dad, do you think I'm fat?"

My father was an extremely caring and loving old school Philadelphian who loved his daughter - his only child - more than he did himself. I am pretty sure he loved me even more than he loved the Philadelphia Eagles.

"Honey, sweetheart, you have the prettiest face in all of Pennsylvania! Don't worry about it."

I knew that meant yes. A pretty face maybe, but fat, absolutely. This is when it started for me. From this point on, the special meals my mom created in the kitchen were not met with comfort, but with avoidance. The kitchen artist started to take offense that her daughter wouldn't eat her food like she used to.

The cycle continued as the years went on. I was never quite thin enough in my eyes, and my mother felt she never could do right anymore by her daughter and responded with mother's guilt.

Over time, my struggle with weight became an obsession, straining almost all the relationships I had fostered over the years. In college I was in and out of relationships that eventually seemed to go south. I was never sure if it was due to my poor self-image or if the relationships just died of natural causes.

After college I met Brad Newman who would become my husband and father of my two boys. He was good to me and consistently told me I do not need to be a certain size. I felt he meant it, but I convinced myself I would not be truly happy until I was the size I felt I needed to be. Skinny.

I had carried this poor self-image since eighth grade. It started with a stupid boy, Devlin Hertz. It was worsened by what my well meaning father said to protect me, and it was intensified by my mother's double helping of guilt and calzone.

Sick and Tired

My discomfort-comfort relationship with food started at age thirteen and continued over the next thirty-two years, right up to this first encounter with Brother Mark, twelve years ago. The demon of a poor self-image possessed me. I chose to believe the lies of the demon who had been whispering in my ear since middle school. He whispered, "You are incomplete."

I could not feel accepted the way I was. The seed of insecurity was planted and it grew and choked out a large part of who I was to become over the next thirty-two years. This understanding became crystal clear on my first encounter with my wise old monk friend. He brought this pain out of me. I don't know how he did it but the tremendous shame I was feeling took me over. It all came to a head on that particular morning a dozen years ago.

"Thirty-two years!" I remember saying out loud, "My God, thirty-two years!"

I thought of the time I spent yo-yo dieting and the money I spent chasing down the path towards the next cure. I thought of the thousands of dollars I had spent over the last decades wrestling with my demon - buying diet books, appetite suppressants, and prescription diet pills without one thought of the money. I thought of the billion people on the planet who could not afford to eat at all, while I poured my resources into unhealthy false hopes to stop over-eating.

The guilt and shame boiled up inside at that halfway point of my first meeting with Brother Mark. I could not control it anymore. I was truly sick to my stomach with emotions!

A weakened heart!

Hypertension, depression, and borderline diabetes!

The diet pills and prescription medications!

The diet books!

Nearly a billion starving!

I was just hacking at leaves!

I remember crying out, "How many mouths could I have fed?"

"What?" the startled monk said to me as he was climbing to his feet. "Are you alright Hope?"

All I remember saying to him was, "I'm sorry...I have to go get some air!"

I rushed out the door of the library, turned the corner and hung my head over the waist high stone fence surrounding the monastery grounds. There, I threw-up everything that was in my stomach.

Part II
STRIKING AT THE ROOT

Hearing Silence

I remember imagining what Brother Mark probably thought of me at that point. I felt at the time he must be thinking I was a real *whack-job*. But, to my surprise he didn't think of me that way at all. In a way, maybe it was part of the process of my rebirth. I had to get rid of everything - hit bottom - before I could receive the education that saved my life. I guess it was a lot like an exorcism. I had to cast out my demon who whispered in my ear for thirty-two years in order to hear the other softer voice.

When Brother Mark finally came outside for me, all I remember doing was apologizing.

"Don't apologize" he said. "I understand how you feel."

Somehow I felt he really did understand. He gestured with his hand towards a new foot path leading from the library to a barn off in the distance at the center of the beautifully colored fields of vegetation. It was a path I didn't notice before.

"Maybe we should just go for walk. I would love to show you the rest of the monastery," he added, "There is so much this place can teach you."

I allowed myself to be effortlessly hoisted to my feet by that eighty-eight year old monk. As we walked together on the new path, I could not help but once again think, *"This old guy is really strong."*

A beautifully red painted barn - typical color barn for this part of Pennsylvania - was several hundred feet up the path through the fields. As we walked towards it in silence, I remember marveling once again at how big the grounds were inside the monastery walls.

I had many questions - so many questions - I would have loved to ask, but felt it would be *unholy* in some way to break the silence.

The silence.

I could not stop thinking about how profound the silence was. I realized that I never made time for *it*.

"It?"

I remember contemplating "it." Was "it" something that was speaking to me inside the solitude? "It" was spiritual, whatever "It" was.

Was "it"...God?

Could God be Who I wasn't hearing when the chatter of life covered up the solitude? That must be it, I remember thinking to myself. God must speak in silence! So I asked Brother Mark point blank, "Does God speak to us in silence?"

"That has been my experience," was his reply.

He told me about the prophet *Elijah* in the Bible and how he heard God's voice as a *still small voice.* He did not hear God in the noisy earthquake, or fire, or hurricane; but in the stillness that followed the storms.

"I guess we all have storms in our lives," I remember saying.

"Yes, it is true, but we will not find God in our storms," he said. "We will find Him in the solitude that follows, when we allow ourselves to *be still.*"

I had experienced that *still small voice* a couple times that morning. Silence had allowed me to face painful memories head on. Silence allowed me to confront my demon.

I learned we can't have peace until we discipline ourselves enough to *be still* and listen. When we don't take time for silence, or stillness, or prayer, or meditation, or whatever you want to call it; we can easily let God's voice be drowned out in the splashing of the shallow end of the swimming pool of life. The shallow end is noisy. The demon spends his time splashing in the shallow end. Still waters run deep. What Brother Mark taught me twelve years ago while walking with him on that new path was this: *God is heard in stillness.*

Deep Water

We also talked about what we learn in *stillness* about *movement.* I thought it was ironic that in *stillness* we get a deeper appreciation for *movement.* It sounds like a contradiction, but what Brother Mark was talking about was the balance between *stillness of the mind* and *movement of the body.*

Over the next hour, Brother Mark taught me how modern conveniences had made our lives sedentary. Our work had advanced from physical to stationary, while our remote controls and drive-thru fast foods had given us little reason to move at all. The irony is, even though we are more sedentary, our bodies still crave movement. That is how we were created to be. We were built to move, to be physical, very physical, yet *progress* tends to lead us more and more towards inactivity.

In a time span where our food was getting more caloric, our bodies were burning fewer calories. The combination had become disastrous for most people. I learned that unlike anything we create by hand which starts to breakdown when used, like a car or a refrigerator, the body improves in every way with moderate to heavy use. Exercise is a magic pill, a fountain of youth, an anti-depressant. The body is improved in every way possible, naturally with exercise.

I remember the monk asking me *how* I exercised. I responded that I was not consistent but had access to a treadmill, a stationary bike, a gym membership. I told him when time allowed, I always tried to work out but often I was too busy.

He asked again, *"How* do you exercise?"

A little confused, I responded a second time. This time I started to tell him about some of the exercises that I usually did whenever I went to the gym, the weights that I used, the repetitions I did.

He wasn't satisfied. He said "I don't mean to sound redundant or disrespectful Hope, but *how* do you exercise?"

That was the third time he asked. I was confused at that point, to be honest. I simply told him that I didn't know what he meant by *how*. Brother Mark was obviously fishing in deeper waters for a bigger answer. He knew I had only been exposed to the noisy shallow side of exercise. I had not yet experienced exercise's true depth.

"Sorry Hope. My question was a trap," he said, "I thought you might have answered the way you did. You answered the question the way you have been *conditioned* to exercise."

I did not know what he meant, but he went on to explain that society had been conditioned to view exercise through a simple *emotional* lens. During the time we were veering away from the whole unprocessed foods that had been provided for us through nature, we had also been unconsciously losing our perspective on the true value and meaning of exercise.

He explained there was a time when being "fit" quite literally could have meant being a better provider for loved ones. Farming a few generations back was a very physical livelihood, and the great majority of people were responsible for raising their own food. Exercise was never thought of, yet everyone did it. The stronger you were and the better your endurance, the more you could plow, plant, and harvest to provide for yourself and others. He said you could still see this physical labor today at the monastery and around the valley at the Amish farms. The Amish do not deal with the same chronic health issues that the people of the modern age do. Their long days are filled with very physical work and they eat the very healthy whole foods they grow. This is the same for the people of Okinawa. Their days are physical and their food is healthy, just like in America a few generations ago.

In the modern age, exercise is thought of emotionally more than ever, yet we are at the most sedentary point in history. Very few people get the full physical benefits of an active lifestyle. We have spent more in recent years on medications, surgeries, and adaptive equipment for chronic conditions that are largely avoidable through the benefits of exercise. Brother Mark taught me that the single most important step we can take as a nation to secure our national healthcare programs is to start eating healthier and exercising faithfully every day. He explained when we understand how exercise helps us more than just reducing weight; it will give us more depth to its real value. It will help us to see exercise as a gift from God, not the chore we made it.

Exercise

One benefit of exercise I was not aware of was how exercise simply helps manage *"arthritis."* Brother Mark explained to me that the *cartilage* is the lining surfaces of any joint, as well as the padding between two bones. Cartilage is what is worn thin with arthritis. He said that cartilage has a poor blood supply and because of this, it doesn't get fed its nutrients as well as muscle because muscle has a good blood supply. Cartilage gets its nutrients from the fluid inside the joint, which is called *synovial* fluid. It is actual movement that allows the joint itself to become nice and flexible and allows the joint to repair itself. It can be compared to working *taffy*. When taffy is cold and dormant, it is hard and brittle; but when you start to move taffy or "exercise" taffy, it becomes nice and pliable.

In addition to helping with arthritis, exercise is also helpful in the prevention of *"osteoporosis."* Most people are aware that osteoporosis leaves the bones more brittle. But, they might not know that exercise causes an increase in the density of bone. The most effective prevention of osteoporosis is a lifetime of exercise.

Brother Mark approached the topic of *"heart disease"* with a little caution to be sympathetic to the diagnosis I was given just before I had the nerve to visit him. He taught me that heart and lung functions are greatly improved with exercise, which improves the oxygen exchange of all the organs; thus improves function and healing of all parts of the body. Exercise does the opposite of smoking. Any destructive habit like smoking not only compromises breathing and makes exercise difficult, but it can also negatively affect any healing that is needed in the body.

The more you improve your heart, lungs, and blood vessels through exercise and not smoking, the better the body works. I remember him looking at my cardiogram and saying I have an excellent chance of strengthening my heart with exercise. This was music to my ears.

The shame is that many people like me needed a diagnosis before they got the message. The greatest tragedy is when people get the warning signs or the diagnosis and still decide that their current unhealthy sedentary lifestyle is perfectly acceptable. They rely only on medication.

Other conditions like *high blood pressure,* also called *hypertension,* can be prevented with exercise over time. Since high blood pressure is really excessive tension in the blood vessels throughout the body, then it makes sense that the stronger or more efficient the heart contracts, the more blood pushes through the body more efficiently with each heartbeat. Thus, in between heart beats, there is less pressure on the blood vessels at rest. Stronger hearts have less constant pressure on the blood vessels throughout the body. Ongoing exercise works like magic in reducing high blood pressure. Remember, exercise is like pressure cleaning your body from the inside. All systems benefit with exercise.

Stress is also a risk factor for high blood pressure. We have a heightened sensitivity in times of stress. This is important when we are in danger, but many times it is chronically self inflicted by our chosen lifestyle of stress.

When we are stressed, blood flow is restricted to our digestive system to allow more blood for our muscles. Among other things, stress causes an increase in blood pressure and heart rate. Many times, if stress is a way of life, one becomes at risk for digestive problems, disturbed sleeping patterns, even a stroke or heart attack. You can see the importance "silence" plays in calming anxiety, worry, or stress.

Excessive body-fat puts more pressure on the heart to pump. The less body-fat one has, the less pressure one has on the heart and blood vessels when pumping the blood through the body.

Even with all these reasons to exercise with a diagnosis of high blood pressure, many people continue to live a life of stress, unhealthy eating, and rely on chemicals to control their health. Unfortunately, when the warning signs like high blood pressure are ignored, grave results can occur. High blood pressure and heart disease can be precursors to a *"stroke."*

A stroke happens when part of the brain stops having blood circulating to it. This causes that part of the brain to die. There are a few reasons why blood is blocked from getting to areas the brain causing a stroke.

Most often a stroke is caused by plaque building-up and blocking the blood flow inside a blood vessel in the brain. Plaque is made up of cholesterol, fat, calcium, or other substances found in the blood. You can think of plaque as "sediment" in the blood that sticks to the blood vessel walls and potentially chokes off the blood from passing through.

A stroke can also be caused by plaque breaking free from somewhere else and settling in smaller blood vessels in the brain causing that part of the brain to die.

Plaque build-up is accelerated in the blood because of poor diet and unhealthy habits like inactivity and smoking.

If you think about it, the blood just wants to move through the body with the greatest of ease. If there is not much activity or movement, then the heart is not getting exercised and the blood is not circulating well. It is kinda like having stagnant water sitting around. You start to get sediment and it becomes harder to circulate. Inside the blood vessels, freely rushing blood is always better. Exercise causes the blood *not* to be stagnant. Movement is life. Once again, we are pressure washed clean on the inside with exercise.

I remember Brother Mark also sharing with me his thoughts on *diabetes.* He said one of the horrible misfortunes he started to see in his practice in the younger patients was a rapid increase of diabetes. He said only a small percentage of diabetes is from childhood viruses or other conditions beyond our control. Ninety percent of pre-diabetes can be controlled or even reversed with eating healthy and exercising.

The wake-up call is really for those who have very poor diets, who might be overweight and don't exercise. It is this ever growing group who are more at risk for developing diabetes.

One of the clever illustrations I remember Brother Mark showing me about exercise was when we were standing at the animal pens at the monastery. He pointed out three big pigs lying out in the sun, caked in mud, happy and lazy as can be. He explained this was what they did if their needs were met. They were happy just as they were. That was their nature. On the farm, they didn't need to expend any more energy than the bare minimum. Their food was brought to them and they did very little work for it.

"It seems like lately we as a society have evolved into this," Brother Mark said to me - half jokingly, but not really.

"Our real nature is more like that dog over there." He pointed behind the cattle pen where a spindly mid-size mutt was chasing something back and forth on the other side of the fence.

"I see him, looks like he's trying to trap a chipmunk or something," I said.

"His desire is to never be lazy," Brother Mark continued. "His nature is one that is to run even if his food bowl is filled."

"So, what are humans made for, running or being lazy?" I asked half jokingly - but not really, "Are we the dog or the pig?"

"Well, the dog of course," the monk replied. "We are to be physical. We know now that when we do exercise of any kind, our bodies change for the better. In other words, if we ate the right whole foods and exercised consistently, if we spent our days chasing chipmunks, then we would be as God intended for us to be – functioning at our physical best."

He gestured back to the pigs. "Unfortunately, when we eat too much of the wrong things, and lose our desire to be physical, we start to develop chronic conditions like obesity and diabetes. Soon, we become more like the pigs."

I kept thinking back to that simple formula while he was comparing the animals.

Calories in < Calories out = Weight loss

It reminded me that all permanent weight loss hangs on that formula. Success of any diet will boil down to that principle. The calorie intake cannot exceed the calorie output. Simple physiology will dictate that you will gain weight if input is greater than output. This formula does not account for nutrition, though. It is simply the formula that cannot be overlooked when trying to stay healthy.

I also learned that the more muscle you have, the easier it is to burn calories. Adding more muscle will also help you stay disability free as you get older.

I learned that muscles shrink over the years. It is an aging condition called *"Sarcopenia."* Sarcopenia is to the muscles, as osteoporosis is to the bones. It can lead to early disability by keeping an older adult wheelchair bound if too much strength is lost. The good news is that exercise can reverse the effects of sarcopenia.

Exercise even affects *"depression"* in a positive way. Addictive substances like alcohol, cocaine, and tobacco stimulate the areas of the brain which causes cravings. So does exercise once it becomes a healthy disciplined daily routine. Destructive addictive habits are replaced by exercise - the healthy alternative. Exercise stimulates the release of *endorphins* in your brain. These are the chemicals that are released naturally, which function like an anti-depressant. So the more you exercise, the more you desire to exercise and the less depressed you feel.

It is easy to imagine that we were created with these endorphins to increase our desire to keep us active for survival. This craving for more movement probably allowed us to eagerly forage for food years ago. Instead of lying around in a depression with no food, endorphins would have us jump out of bed to find breakfast because we craved food and we craved movement.

Many cancers are also found to be linked directly to our nation's diet and lack of exercise.

As you can see, exercise is so much more than a tool for weight-loss. It is a gift from God for a life of health and wellness. This is the revelation I received that day twelve years ago from Brother Mark on the value of exercise.

Faith & Fitness

At this point in the story that I am sharing with you about the four hours I spent with Brother Mark, I think it is important to explain something more clearly.

Most of what he told me about exercise after I had my crazy mental breakdown in front of him was information that I already knew about exercise, or if I didn't know it, I could have looked it up and found it out for myself. But, that wasn't the important part of the education. The most important lesson I learned was not the details but the big picture Brother Mark drew for me. What he taught me was a new motivation I needed to stay committed to a life of exercise and eating healthy. This is the part of this story I really want you to pay close attention to, especially if you are one of the people who Brother Mark was concerned about. If you are like I was, in desperate need of someone to *catch* you so you don't fall off a cliff of despair, or death, or something – then I pray you get this connection he made for me.

Brother Mark brought to life a much larger and more important reason to commit to a healthy lifestyle. Losing weight is a fleeting goal that is here today and gone tomorrow. It is full of emotion and won't last long. But, *caring for myself so I can better care for others* was that faith and fitness connection I finally understood. It integrated for me food, exercise, and a genuinely happy purposeful life. I waited thirty-two years for that message.

Whole Foods

Nothing that Brother Mark taught me that morning made the connection of faith and fitness more clear then when he explained how God provided and nourished us from nature. He helped me understand the following: Everything we need to sustain life has already been provided to us already, naturally. If this was not true, then life would have never been.

His explanation of what happened when we started to farm the conventional way was the education I needed to hear in order to understand where I personally had gone wrong regarding how I understood food.

He explained the fundamentals of farming changed in many ways since he was a kid. From the mass production of raising *corn*, to the loss of sustainable family farms, to the way livestock was raised - all these changes directly affected the way we eat today. It is completely different than it was a few generations ago.

The new conventional use of fertilizers, pesticides, and insecticides helped to make *corn* the most versatile of all crops. Smaller farms were bought up by bigger ones to more efficiently grow corn. The *efficiency* of food production increased tremendously into the mass production of one golden mega crop, corn.

As the corn bins filled, a surplus started to be accumulated and before long, scientists discovered that there was very little one can't do with corn. It could be turned to alcohol to drink or used as fuel. It could be fed to cattle, chickens, and pigs. Corn could be dried and stored away as long as needed, unlike fresh vegetables that spoil in a short time after picking. This made corn even more a cost effective commodity for the consumer.

Corn was processed to make *high fructose corn syrup* and replaced cane sugar as the sweetener in food, since it could be made more efficiently. In fact, as the processed food industry progressed, one would be hard pressed to find any processed food or soft drink that did not use high fructose corn syrup for sweetener. Breakfast cereals, cooking oils, and even lubricants for skin care, all contained extracted and processed corn.

Cheap meats were made possible primarily due to the feeding of corn to the livestock on feed lots. Brother Mark went on to say that high fructose corn syrup and cheap meats made it easy to have inexpensive processed food available all the time. Today, we can get a hamburger, fries, and a soda anytime and anyplace we want. Food processing made this possible. We can ship processed foods from anywhere to anywhere - our cheap meats for burgers, our potatoes for fries, and high fructose corn syrups for soda. Eating in America has become almost effortless and automated, thanks to the incredible advancement of food processing and thanks primarily to corn.

With that, we are taking in more saturated animal fats and sugar than at anytime in history.

In addition to the unhealthy effects of fast food, conventional mass production farming affects us in indirect ways as well. Brother Mark explained that there are miles of mildly poisoned rivers and river basins largely due to use of fertilizers and insecticides. In conventional growing, where massive corn acreage is replanted each year, more chemical fertilizers are used as necessary to replace lost nitrogen in the topsoil. The runoff from the fertilizers and pesticides is what is poisoning waterways.

The Amish, the monks, the people of Okinawa, and the generations before us all farmed organically, thus returning nitrogen to the soil through biodiversity and crop rotations which rebuilds and preserves the nutrient rich topsoil.

Because of progress, the grazing cattle have become something of the past for many large processing plants. Cattle have been pulled from the pastures - away from grazing - and put into pens on the high density feed lots.

On the feed lots, they eat corn, not naturally growing pasture grasses. When these great animals are huddled together and fed corn - which is digestible but not the natural diet for them - they often develop intestinal problems. This requires antibiotics. In addition, close proximity causes parasites to spread easily from animal to animal. This requires more antibiotics. Feces in the meat can create harmful parasites when ingested by humans.

Cattle have become much less of a valued member of a natural ecosystem on the concentrated cattle operations. Even manure is no longer a useful fertilizer like it used to be when it was distributed evenly in the grazing fields. In such great concentrations on the feed lots, it becomes harmful to neighboring waterways and neighborhoods.

The real crime is that for the first time in history because of excess calories through efficiency, we no longer look at our food as being a blessing but a curse. Because food is so processed, accessible and plentiful, we simply eat the wrong foods and too much of it. Brother Mark taught me today's health crisis is not the fault of the individual, but it is a manifestation of our nation forgetting our blessings of real, whole, natural foods and simple life giving fresh water.

Local, Seasonal, Organic

Brother Mark feels we have abandoned the natural order and timing of our Creator's provisions. Instead, we fed an unsustainable appetite. Unlike the Amish, the monks, the people of Okinawa and the generations before us; we have tampered with the waste free ecosystem that was naturally and perfectly sustainable. Brother Mark taught me that if we stepped out of the way, nature is completely integrated within itself. The rain falls and the grass and plants grow; which are grazed by the herbivores; which are eaten by the carnivores. The carcasses of the herbivores and the carnivores are eventually eaten by the scavengers; then the insects and the worms return the nutrients to the soil. Then rain falls...you get the picture. In nature, there is one big cycle and nothing goes to waste.

On the monk's farm, they had several pens of animals that are rotated. The cattle eat the grass and are rotated into another pen so that the grass can grow again. The chickens come in after the cattle and scratch and pick out the parasites from the dung. I know it sounds unappetizing but they find juicy maggots, bugs, and other larvae in the manure. The chickens love it and the field is now canvassed with natural fertilizer from the cattle and chickens; and the grass can grow stronger and greener, naturally. The cycle repeats itself over and over, and nothing goes to waste. No chemical or artificial fertilizer is needed for the farm. The monks had respectfully integrated themselves into nature. Every animal serves a valuable purpose. It doesn't get more natural, or greener, than that.

When we learn to work with nature, insects that can ruin certain types of fruits and vegetables are not a problem if we also invite their natural predators. Insects do the job that chemical insecticides do, but naturally.

Roles are played out in nature. Nature is in a healthy partnership with all components of itself. Everything has its role to play. If the grass said to the soil *"today I refuse to grow,"* then the grass would not grow, the cows could not graze, the vegetables would be without the cow's fertilizer, and the chickens could not get the grubs that are in the manure as part of their standard diet. When we tamper too much with the rhythms of nature, we change the process of our planet's health, our personal health, and the animals who offer their very lives for our nourishment.

In talking with Brother Mark, I also learned that the average person of wealthy nations like ours produce a total of almost five pounds of trash in a day each. This includes the trash produced to manufacture the packaging of the processed food and drink we consume. It takes a lot of resources behind the scenes to make one ready-made food item.

When we eat directly from the ground, vines, trees, and fields - like the monks on the farm, like the Amish, like the people from Okinawa, and like the generations before us - we create a symbiotic relationship with the earth in which chemicals, processing, additives, and packaging are almost non-existent. When an individual eats mindfully, garbage from the food and beverage packaging can be reduced by 90%.

The more local and seasonal we can learn to eat, the less dependency we will have on oil for transportation, processing, and packaging. Local food eaten in season ultimately can remain fresher and more nutritious longer. The typical consumer has no idea just how much fossil fuels are used in our conventional way of eating. Between producing the fertilizers, pesticides, harvesting, and transporting; modern food production uses about a third of the total fossil fuels we use in this country. To give you an example, it takes about fifty gallons of oil to produce an acre of corn through conventional farming.

If we learn to eat more local, seasonal and organic foods, we would relieve the need for foreign oil, our gasoline costs would greatly reduce, and we would be much healthier as a people and a planet. Thinking local, seasonal, and organic when it comes to our food, keeps nature and our health in balance.

Why don't we all eat this way?

Before Brother Mark taught me how we are so intimately connected to nature, I ate unconsciously and poorly, mostly due to the fact that it is just *easier* and cheaper to eat that way. I suppose it is true for everyone if they are not enlightened to the overall benefits. We don't eat well because it is more convenient to eat poorly.

The same question could be asked with exercise.

Why are we all not exercising if we can reduce obesity, arthritis, osteoporosis, heart disease, high blood pressure, diabetes, sarcopenia, strokes, cancer and depression?

I know we don't exercise for the same reason we don't eat well. We don't exercise because it is more convenient to stay sedentary.

Before my enlightenment with Brother Mark, I only saw one dimension: exercise was a tool for weight-loss and nothing more. Since my awakening, I see all dimensions of exercise. The same is true for the local, seasonal, and organic foods we eat. It is not just trendy or simply healthy for me, it is healthy for the planet which makes it healthy for all of us.

Greatest Desire

The beauty of the monastery will always be fresh in my memory. I can't think of a place so immense in size yet offered such simple and plain charm. I can remember vividly when our four hours were coming to an end. There was a moment when the faith and fitness connection was most self-evident. It was when Brother Mark and I climbed the stone steps to the top of the chapel and looked over the entire monastery.

From this view, I could see the whole property was the size of maybe six or seven football fields put side by side to make one giant rectangle. The farm in the center of the property took up most of the acreage. Surrounding the farm in each corner of the rectangle were the four stone buildings: the *refectory* or dining hall, the library, the living quarters where the monks slept, and the chapel where we stood above it all. Just to the outside of all of it, the stone waist high fence enclosed the monastery in completely.

The farm was broken up into sections of pens and gardens with wooden fencing. One pen housed those three pigs, and another had sheep, and another had a large portable hen house. In a half dozen different pens were colorful vegetable gardens of every shade of green you can imagine. There were cattle in three other pens, and goats in another. Two monks were guiding a cow carefully from one pen to another with a simple wooden stick. Everywhere I looked I saw green set against the brown fence boards and the dark brown robes of the monks in various pens. There were white, black and brown spots speckled on the animals;

and in the center of it all was that beautiful red barn. I could see all the paths we walked on.

From the view I had from above, I saw how all the paths were connected. I could not see the connection from below. From below, I was only partially aware; I could only see one path at a time. From above, I could see how it all fit together perfectly.

There were dazzling sunflowers, marigolds, and various assortments of flowers peppered yellow and gold throughout the green gardens. They were used for pollination and natural insecticides.

The sun was directly over-head at that point at the end of our time together. The breeze was cool and light. I will never forget it. I was transformed by nature's beauty.

It was about that time when Brother Mark decided to hit me with the big and final question. He asked "Hope, what do you feel is the greatest desire of all people?"

I was intrigued. I was surprised in forty-five years I never asked myself that question.

Money? Is that what people desire most?   Nope, too small, I thought.

"Food, Shelter, Clothing?" No.

"Career?" Important, but still there has to be more.

"Health?" Maybe.

Everything I came up with just seemed too small.

"What is the greatest desire of all people?" I pondered the question as I was taking in the landscape.

Meanwhile, Brother Mark quickly disappeared into the chapel and came back with an old leather bound tattered Bible. I hardly noticed his absence. I was too deeply contemplating his question. I was too busy admiring the painted colors of nature.

Brother Mark opened the Bible to the first few pages of Genesis and read aloud: *God said, 'I give you every seed-bearing plant on the face of the whole earth and every tree that has fruit with seed in it. They will be yours for food. And to the beasts of the earth and all the birds of the air and all the creatures that move on the ground-everything that has the breath of life in it-I give every green plant for food.' And it was so. God saw all that he had made, and, it was very good. (Genesis 1:29-31, NIV)*

I remember a clear thought hit me about what he just finished reading. Maybe it was the combination of the last four hours and the majestic surroundings of nature, but it occurred to me that I was still connected to God through all those years walking the dimly lit path I chose. God clearly had provided for me, or else I simply...well...I simply wouldn't be alive at all. He created me. He did not have to. He chose to. He cared for me all along regardless of whether I was aware of His presence or not. God provided for me everything I needed to be healthy and well, and He said it was good! I just could not hear His *still small voice* during the dark years, there was simply too much chatter from the demon of my poor self image. All of my unhappiness was just me hopelessly striking at leaves in the dark; at the root was genuine happiness all along. At the root was light.

I knew the ultimate lesson Brother Mark was driving at over the four hours that morning. It was our greatest desire: *to be genuinely happy.* I remember my eyes began to fill with tears at my epiphany. I began to see light.

If we feel God loves and provides for us along the path we travel, we will experience interconnectedness with the lives of others and the world we live in. We will know our life matters since it matters to the very One who brought us into existence and sustains us throughout our journey. We will know life matters for others as well. Our happiness will come from within. If we have full awareness of this, then we will be genuinely happy in every endeavor and season of life while giving thanks for the provisions we receive. We will be inspired to share those provisions. Since we matter and others matter, then we will *care for ourselves to better care for others.*

Likewise, if we feel unloved and alone in our journey, we might try to mask our pain with drugs and alcohol, abusive relationships, comfort food, or maybe even starvation or bingeing. We might wander aimlessly battling for acceptance, trying to reinvent ourselves into someone lovable, because who we are seems incomplete and unworthy of genuine love. Since we can only be who we were created to be, we will never have genuine happiness from within. We will only experience temporary moments of fleeting happiness that is dependent on external circumstances: the weather, the paycheck, and the scale.

I turned to face Brother Mark. My eyes were filled with tears, again. Although I was uncontrollably crying off and on most of that morning, I could sense he knew these were happy tears. Before I even spoke I could tell he sensed my awakening.

"What do people deeply desire most of all whether they are aware of it or not?" I restated the question to Brother Mark, *"To be genuinely happy. Once someone knows they are loved by God just the way they are and not as they think they should be; then they will find meaning in the one life they have been given and they will truly and genuinely be happy."

I remember Brother Mark smiling, nodding, and embracing me with a big hug. At that moment of clarity, after sinking as low as I could go so I could be reconstructed by God's grace - I knew after four hours - the student had absorbed the timeless wisdom of the master. For the first time in thirty-two years, I was genuinely happy.

Better

I was saved that day twelve years ago. Not just physically, but mentally and spiritually as well. I finally felt secure in the way God created me.

When we are secure in ourselves then we can *care for ourselves to better care for others* and all our efforts made towards personal fitness can become a true spiritual discipline, an expression of gratitude and thanksgiving for all of life. True wellbeing starts there. It is all about *grace*. That is, it is all about God's free and unmerited favor. He graces us with real food. He graces us with the gift of exercise. His grace is sufficient. We can simply be content in knowing this. We can be genuinely happy. In the presence of God's grace, there are no demons.

A week after the meeting that changed my life, I was down two pounds, four, six, and then ten pounds after the first month. After another month, I lost a total of twenty pounds. Six months after my first encounter with Brother Mark, I was down forty pounds of body fat and I felt I was at a good place. I wasn't skinny. I was healthy. I felt good. I ate right. I gave thanks often. I was mindful of the less fortunate. My exercise routine was a consistent six mile run every day along with a few days a week of weight training. It is still my routine.

In psychology there is a phenomenon called "Flow" that happens when someone becomes totally absorbed in a meaningful task at hand. Time stands still. It is as if one is in an elevated euphoric state of mind. It is similar to "Runner's High". Runner's High happens when someone exercises with consistency over time. You can think of it as your restless mind and spirit being stilled by the rhythmic movement of your body. In other words, there is *stillness* of the mind with *movement* of the body. You find yourself in a new place of solitude while exercising. Some runners say they feel God's presence on the path next to them.

After six months of running, I finally hit that "high." I entered that "Flow" of mind and body. It was an experience I had never had before. I never exercised consistently enough in the past to benefit from this ongoing endorphin rush. Now my daily exercise is effortless. I crave it now. God has been with me on the path ever since.

Running makes me feel better. Eating healthy makes me feel better. I like to feel this way everyday.

One year since that four hour visit with Brother Mark, upon my yearly check-up with the cardiologist, it was discovered that I was on the mend. The weakened heart I was diagnosed with was in fact getting stronger. There was much less strain from obesity. There was no sign of borderline diabetes and no high blood pressure. My body and blood was moving more efficiently. I was getting better. I certainly wasn't depressed anymore.

Each yearly check-up after, my health just kept getting better.

Life Now

I am finally getting to the end of what my mentor and friend Brother Mark wanted me to write. I guess you can tell why, after twelve years, I still consider Brother Mark my *Catcher,* like the Holden Caulfield character in *The Catcher in the Rye.* He caught me from falling off the cliff. And I hope my story will catch you before you fall off the cliff; that is if you are one of those people who Brother Mark was worried about. If you are one of those people, I am glad you heard my story.

At the very time I am writing this, a dozen years have passed since those four hours that changed my life forever. I am now fifty-seven and Brother Mark is a healthy one-hundred years old. Thank God.

On Brother Mark's 100th birthday, hundreds of us pupils who were "caught" by him, threw him a surprise birthday party. It was big news. He was touted as the most famous *centenarian* or one-hundred year old in the valley by all the admirers and students he helped over the twenty-five years.

The party was at the monastery, the very place where I was restored by the grace of God in four hours.

Even though he is now quite famous, my one-hundred year old monk friend will not bother with the attention. He continues to enjoy what he does best: farming, reading, and dispensing his legendary message one hopeful visitor at a time like he has done for twenty-five years. He knows one day that he will not be around and that doesn't bother him. Not one bit. He knows he will have left this planet much better off. He knows his life has deep meaning. He is genuinely happy.

Who knows, maybe with the seeds he planted, the rest of us will carry on his mission and bring in a big harvest and make this a well planet once again. Then humanity will no longer be hacking at the leaves when it comes to health and wellness; but instead, humanity will strike at the root.

That is my story. Thanks for listening and be well. Your Catcher, Hope.

The Faith & Fitness Collection

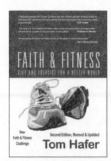

Faith & Fitness
Diet and Exercise for a Better World
Tom Hafer
Huff Publishing Associates, 2014

When we learn to care for ourselves to better care for others we simplify and intensify our quest towards personal fitness. This is the spiritual journey of Faith & Fitness.

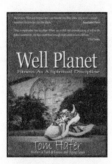

Well Planet
Fitness as a Spiritual Discipline
Tom Hafer
Huff Publishing Associates, 2015

Timeless wisdom for everyone who has fought the demons of weight-loss and won, then lost, then gained, then lost. For the sake of our personal health, our neighbor, and the planet; we have never had a timelier message to embrace...once again.

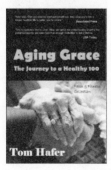

Aging Grace
The Journey to a Healthy 100
Tom Hafer
Huff Publishing Associates, 2014

Explore the "thin place" where the physical and the spiritual worlds are paper thin. Discover the life patterns of real people, who have loved 100 healthy and inspired years of living.

www.tomhafer.com

Join Us

Sundays at 11:00 a.m.
Eastern Time

www.voa.org/worship

Our online worship experience. Leading the worship is Pastor Tom
Hafer, author of *Faith & Fitness, Wellplanet,* and *Aging Grace.*